WHAT HAPPENS

a kid has

cancer

written + illustrated by
SARA OLSHER

Hi, my name is Mia!

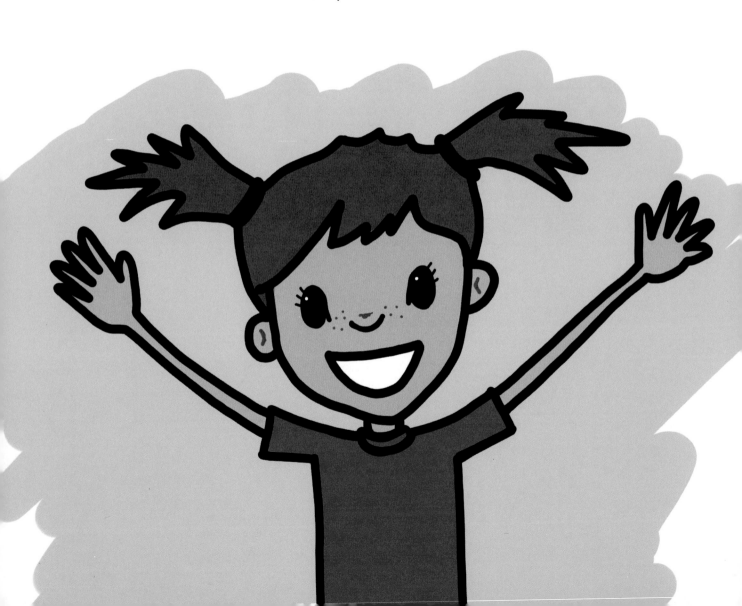

And this is Stuart.
Stuart feels better when he knows
what's going to happen every day.

(Actually, *everybody* feels better when they know
what's going to happen—even grown-ups!)

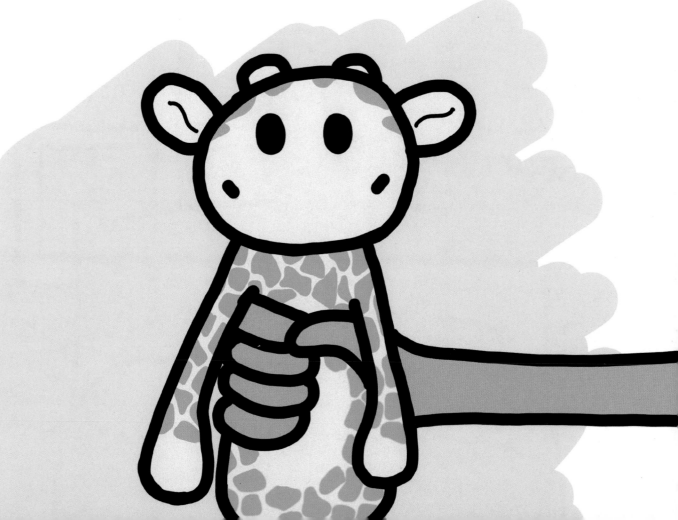

Most of the time,
we do the same things in the mornings.
We wake up.

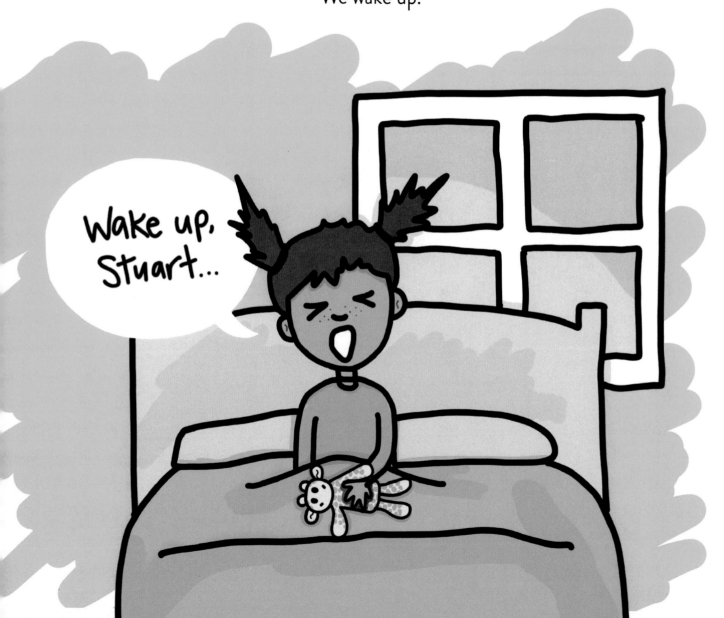

We eat breakfast.
(I like apples. Stuart only eats bugs.)

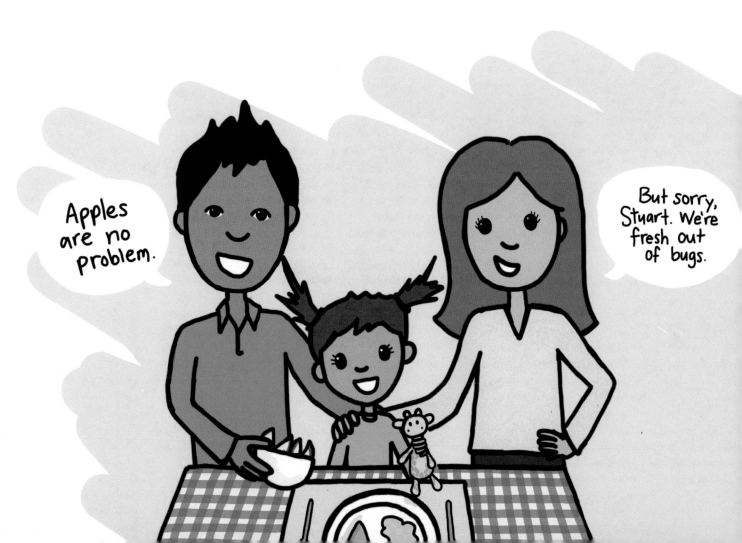

Usually our nights are the same too.
We brush our teeth.

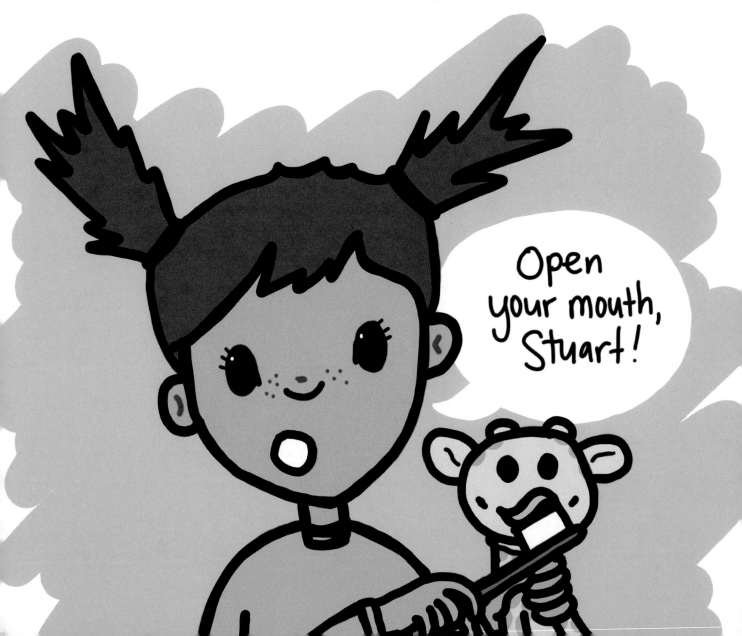

We put on our jammies, and we go to bed.
Every day ends with sleep.

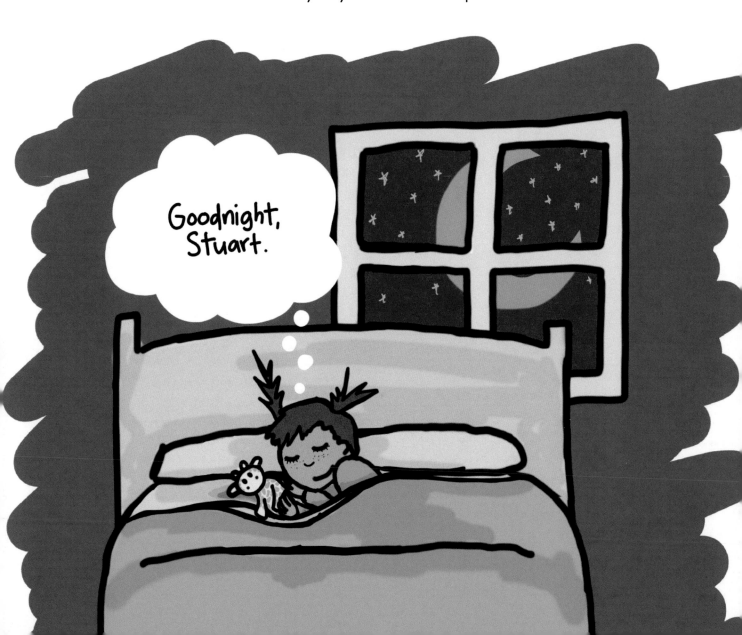

But our days can be different.

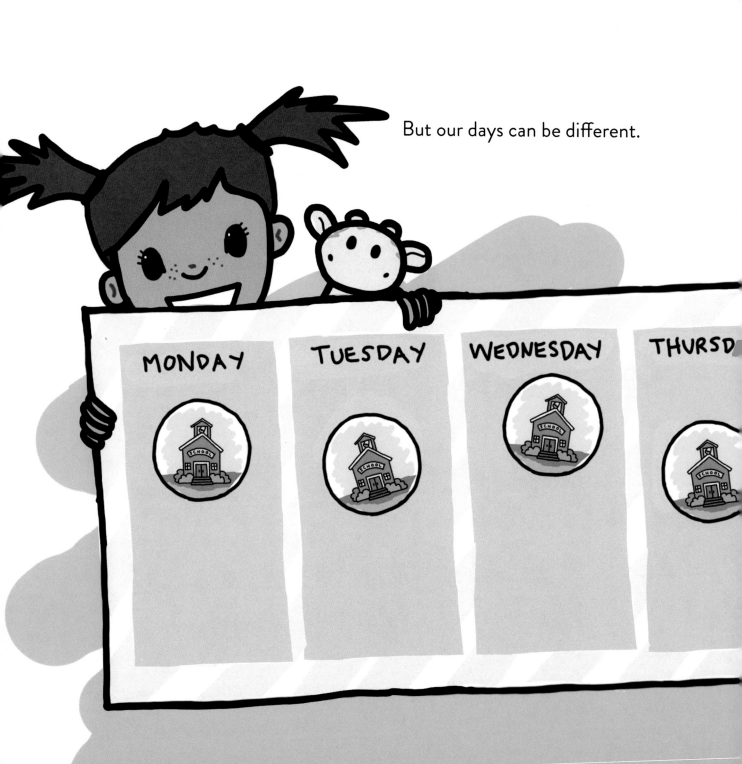

Some days we go to school,
and some days are the weekend!

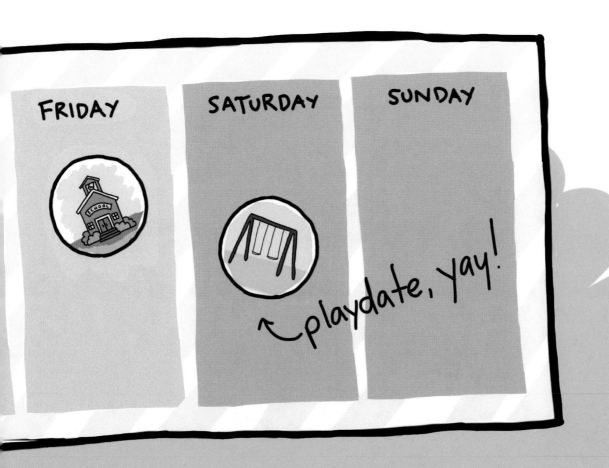

When something big changes,
what we do each day can change too.
Stuart wants to know what happens to our days
when we have **cancer**.

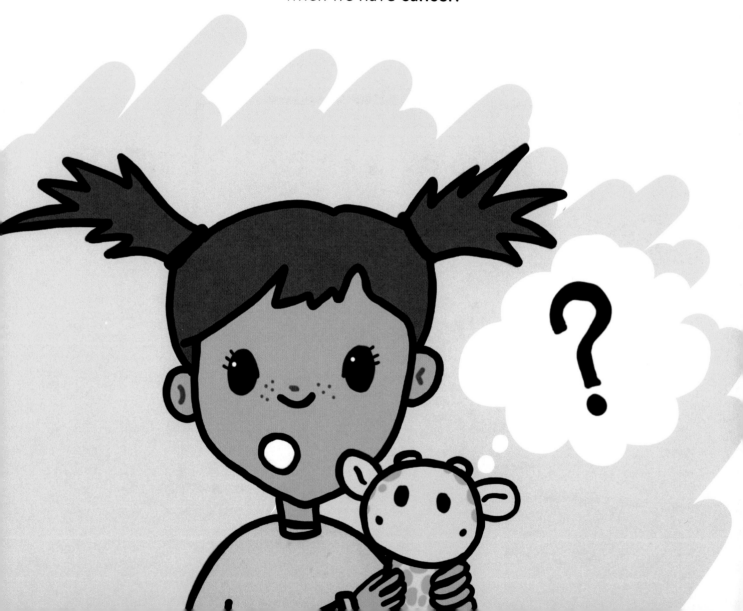

But he doesn't really understand what cancer is. Do you?
Cancer is sort of like a sickness,
but you can't catch it like you catch a cold.

Here's how it works!

Every living thing is made up of tiny little guys called **cells**.

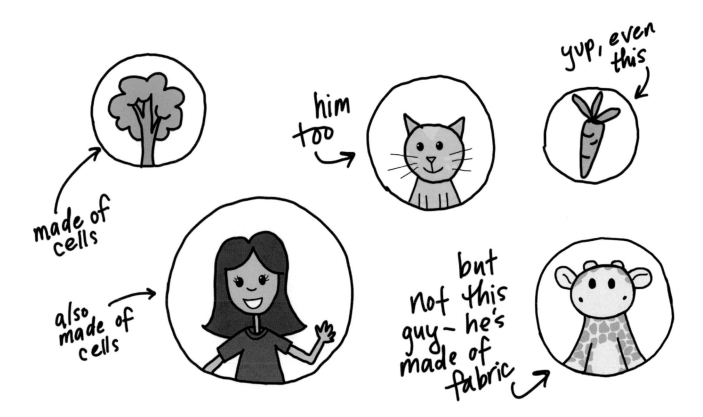

Cells are like blocks, but they put *themselves* together.
One really cool thing about cells is that one cell can
turn itself into two cells anytime it wants.
(*Whoa*, right?)

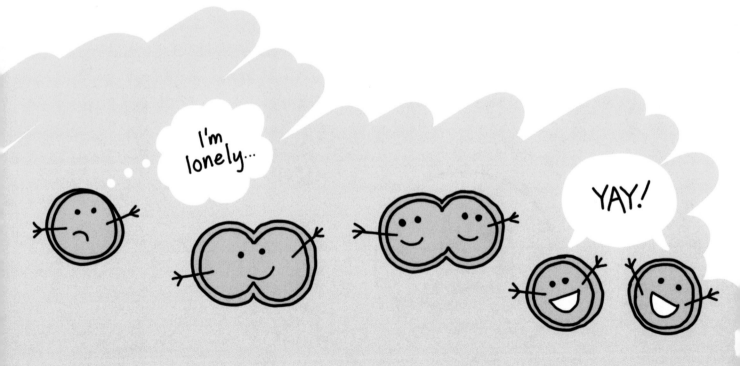

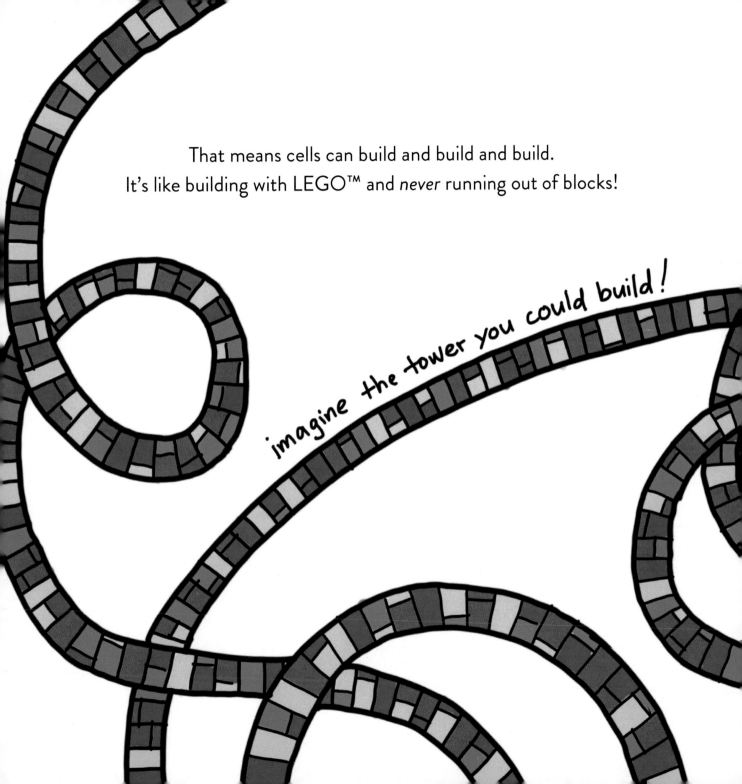

That means cells can build and build and build.
It's like building with LEGO™ and *never* running out of blocks!

imagine the tower you could build!

Every cell has a job.
Together they build body parts, then tell them how to work.
They make hearts pump, legs walk, lungs breathe,
and so much more!

Cells are very polite.
They give each other space to work,
and they stop making new cells when they have enough to do a job.

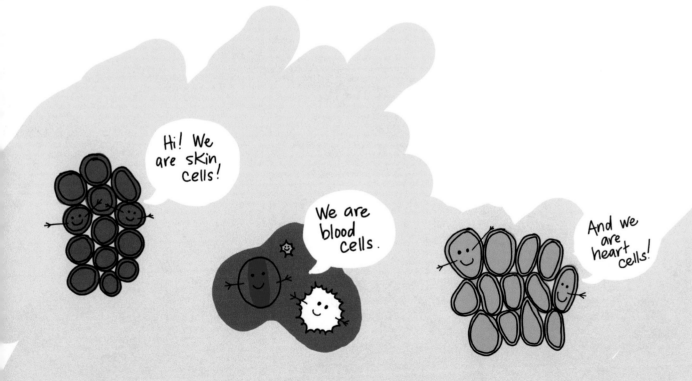

But sometimes a broken cell gets made.
It looks weird, acts weird, and doesn't know what its job is.
The only thing it remembers how to do is make more cells.

Nobody caused this cell to break.
It wasn't anything the person ate or did wrong! Sometimes cells break.

And one or two broken cells is no big deal,
because our healthy cells can get rid of them.
But sometimes the healthy cells don't see the broken cells ...

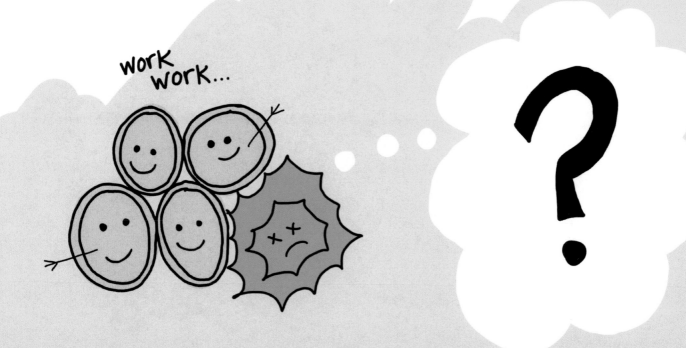

work
work...

... and the broken cells keep making
more and more broken cells, faster and faster.

Before long, it's a *huge* mess.
This huge mess of broken cells is called cancer.

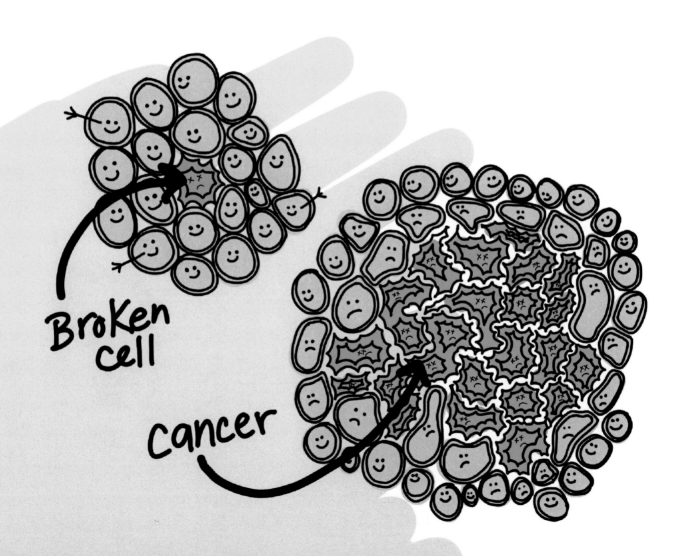

Broken
cell

cancer

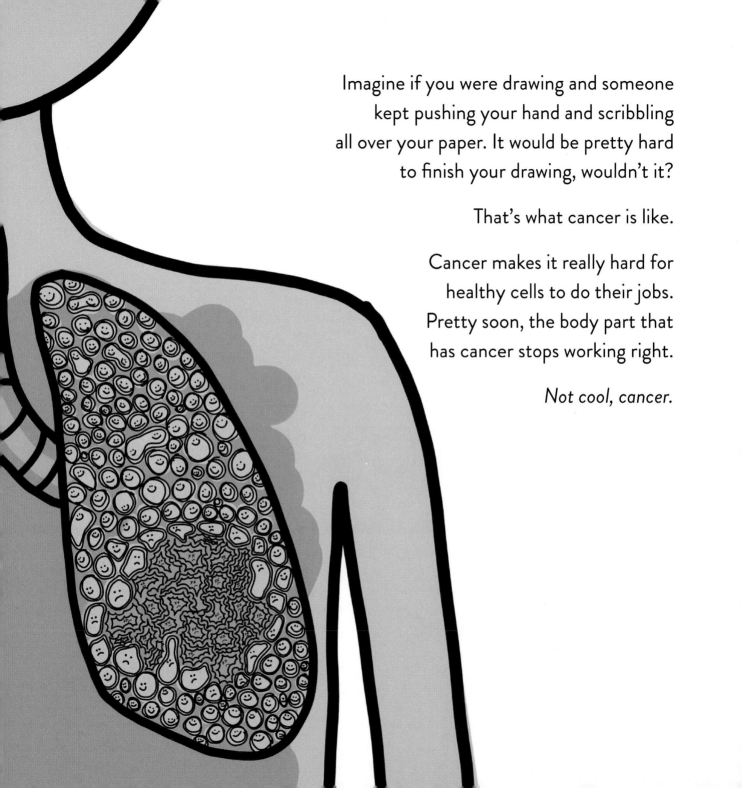

Imagine if you were drawing and someone kept pushing your hand and scribbling all over your paper. It would be pretty hard to finish your drawing, wouldn't it?

That's what cancer is like.

Cancer makes it really hard for healthy cells to do their jobs. Pretty soon, the body part that has cancer stops working right.

Not cool, cancer.

When our healthy cells get crowded by cancer,
they aren't able to do their jobs.
And if they can't do their jobs, our bodies might not work right.

So when someone finds cancer in their body,
they definitely want to get it out.

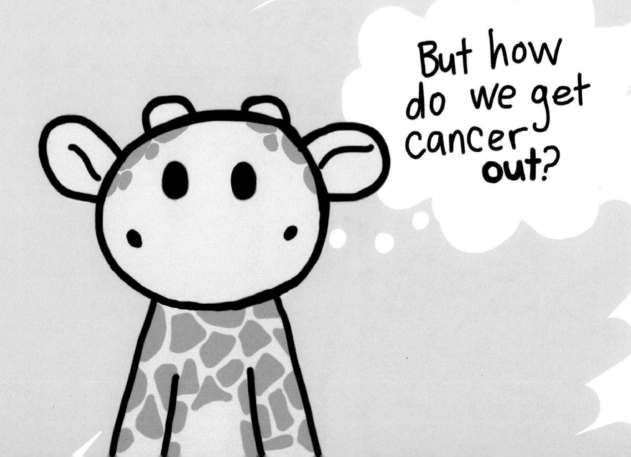

But how do we get cancer out?

Some cancer cells live in blood, and some cancer cells live in body parts.
Doctors can take some types of cancer cells out
of a person's body by giving them surgery.

This means the doctors will give you a medicine
that makes you sleepy called **anesthesia**.
Sometimes you get the sleepy medicine through a special mask.

Then they carefully take out the broken cells.
Because you are sleeping, you don't feel anything!

And when you wake up, your family will be there.

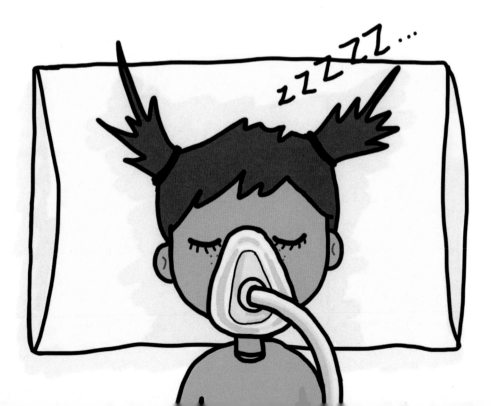

Doctors might also give you a medicine called **chemo**,
which kills cancer cells.
Some days you might need to go to the hospital
or a doctor's office to get chemo.

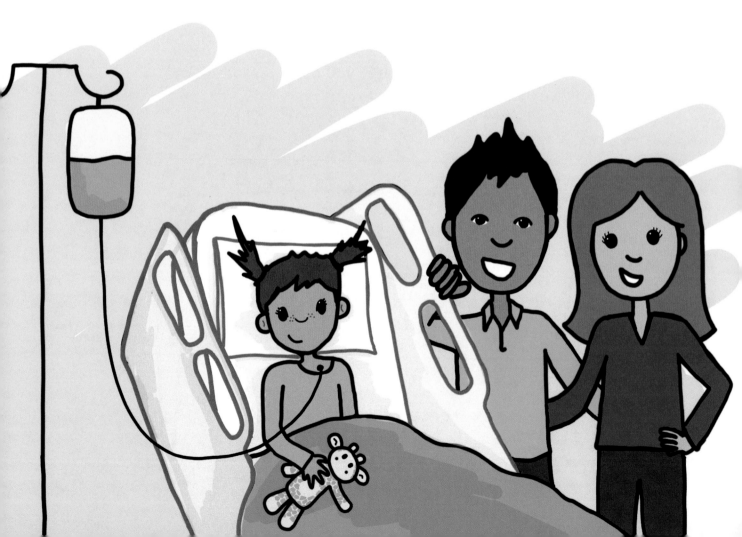

The chemo medicine is super strong and destroys the broken cells,
but it isn't super smart. It also destroys some of the good cells.

Because of this, chemo can make you feel tired.
It might also make your tummy ache or the inside of your mouth hurt.

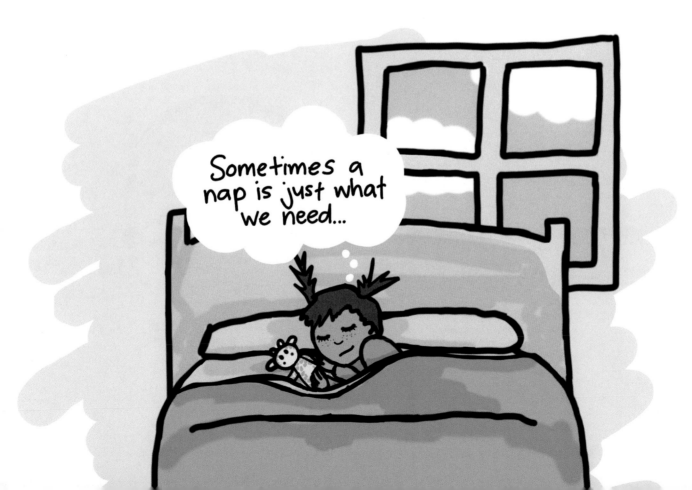

Chemo sometimes also kills the cells that create hair,
which can make your hair fall out.

Some kids lose a little bit of their hair. Some lose lots or all of it.
And some kids don't lose their hair at all.

But don't worry. When chemo is over, the hair will grow back.

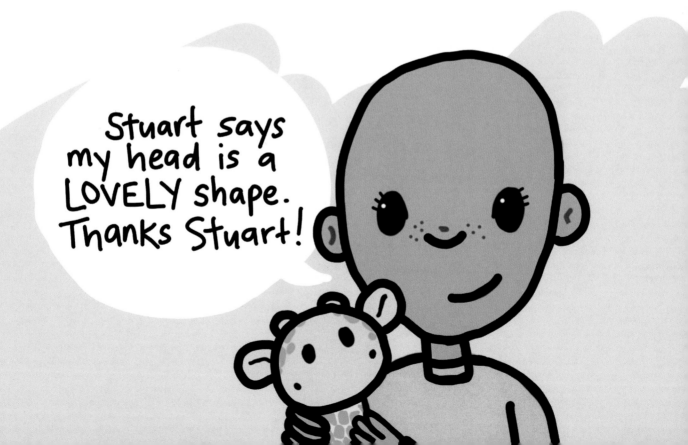

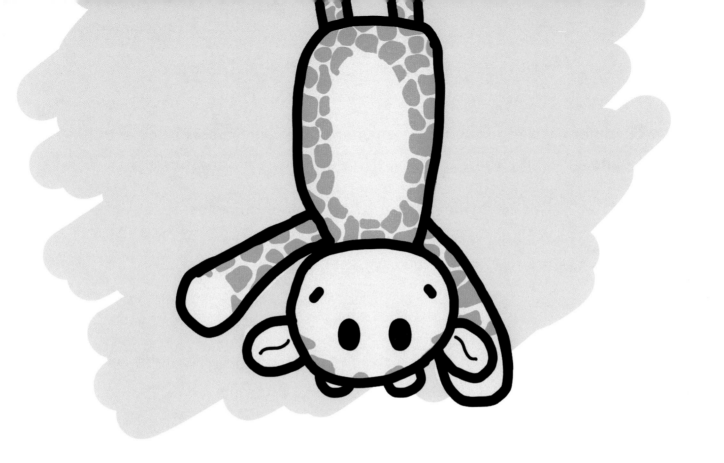

Stuart wants to know what else might happen.

The answer is different for every kid!

But you should tell your family
if your body is feeling different, like if your tummy hurts.

You might have a special button on your chest called a **port** or a **central line**, which is a thin, soft tube that goes into your chest or arm.

This will make it easier to get chemo medicine
and any other medicine you might need
to make you feel better.

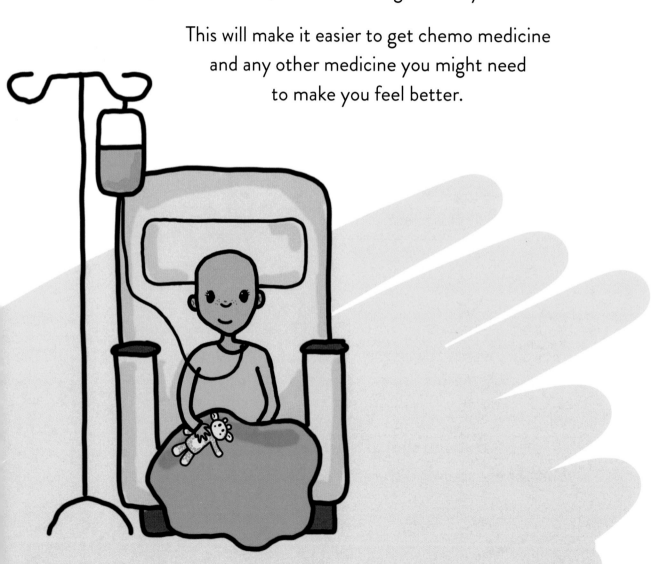

Sometimes you might need to sleep at the hospital
so the doctors and nurses can help you feel better.

Stuart can come, and there's a bed for
a grown-up who loves you too.
You won't be alone.

Plus, the hospital for kids has a playroom, lots of games and toys,
and screen time. Other kids are there who are
getting rid of their cancer too.

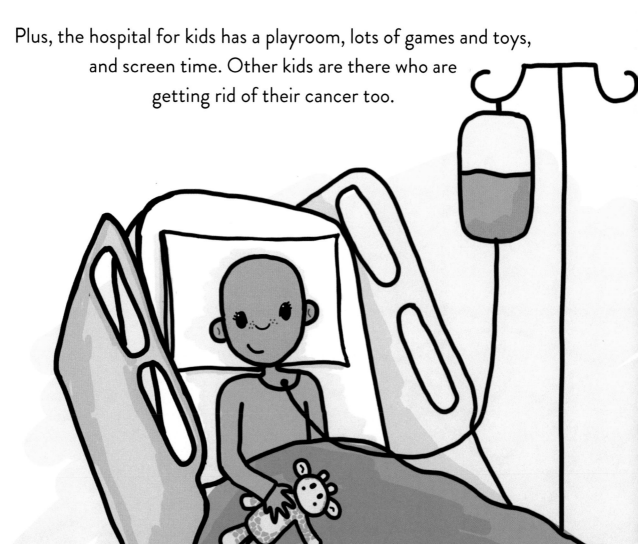

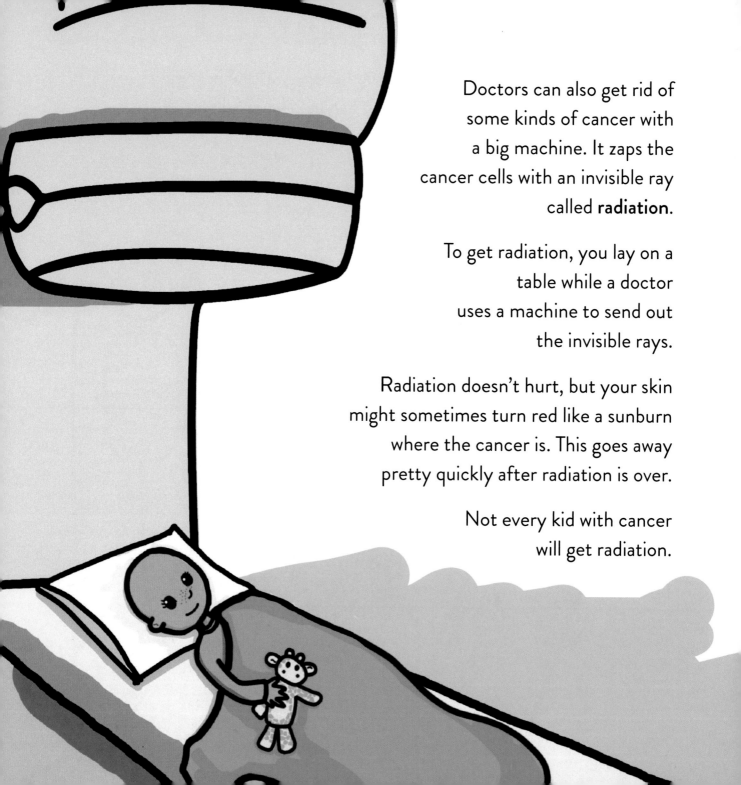

Doctors can also get rid of some kinds of cancer with a big machine. It zaps the cancer cells with an invisible ray called **radiation**.

To get radiation, you lay on a table while a doctor uses a machine to send out the invisible rays.

Radiation doesn't hurt, but your skin might sometimes turn red like a sunburn where the cancer is. This goes away pretty quickly after radiation is over.

Not every kid with cancer will get radiation.

Sometimes the doctors want to know whether the medicines are working. They can do this in two ways.

One way is by taking a picture using a big machine. This is called a **scan**. The scan helps doctors see what the broken cells are doing inside your body.

The other way is by checking your blood to see how many broken cells are hiding. This is called a **blood draw**.

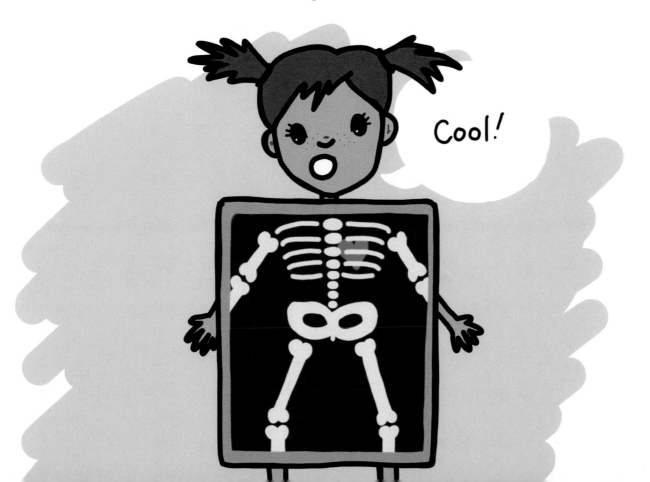

Every kid's cancer is different,
so not every kid will have chemo, radiation, or surgery.
Your doctor and family can tell you what you can expect.

But one thing is true for every kid's cancer:
You didn't make it happen (that's impossible).
And unfortunately, there's nothing you can do
to make it go away all by yourself.

The good news is, once you understand what it's going to be like,
it gets way less scary.

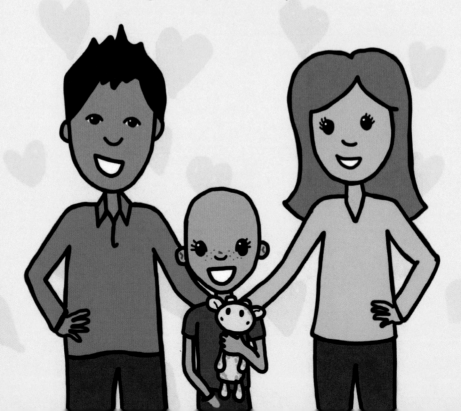

Plus, all the time in the hospital is worth it when the cancer cells are gone and your body has some time to feel better.

All the cells are doing their jobs, and the body is healthy again.
And you know what that means?

A healthy body that can run, jump, swim, and play again
... and grow new hair!

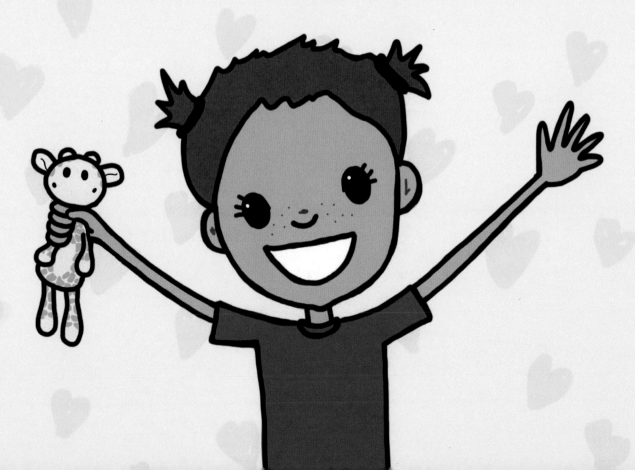

Stuart feels a lot better now that he knows what to expect.

Even though our days can be different,
it helps to plan out our week together,
so we know what's going to happen next.

We can see when our appointments are
and give ourselves activities to look forward to,
like making crafts, watching a movie, or being outside.

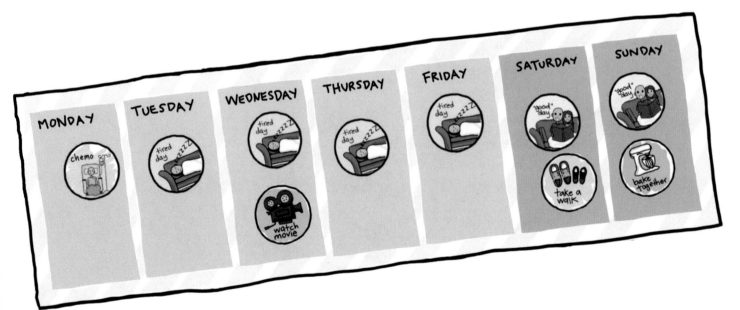

And remember that it's important to share
how you are feeling with a grown-up.
All these changes can be hard!

By planning special time together,
you have a time when you know it's okay to talk about your feelings.
We can do hard things—together!

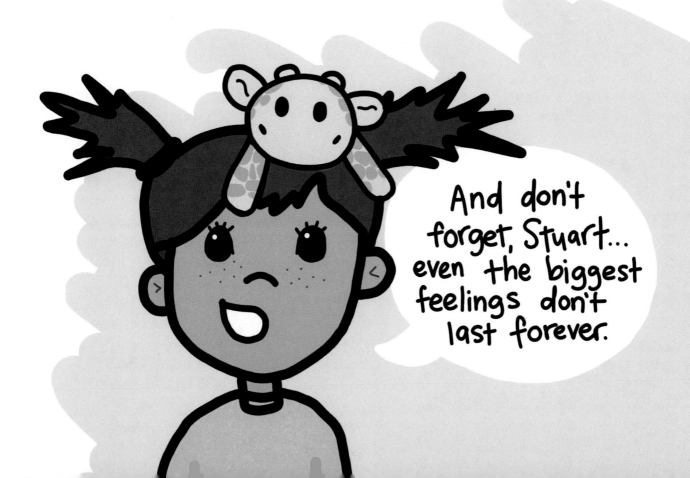

And don't forget, Stuart... even the biggest feelings don't last forever.

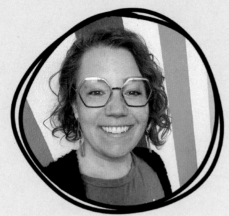

Hi! my name is Sara, and I had cancer, too.

I wrote this book (and 6 others!) because I like to draw + help people.

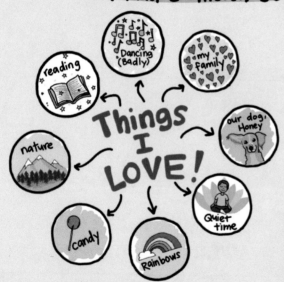

reading

Dancing (Badly)

my family

nature

Things I LOVE!

our dog, Honey

candy

Rainbows

Quiet time

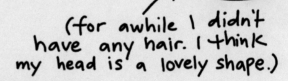

(for awhile I didn't have any hair. I think my head is a lovely shape.)

I live with my daughter, my partner, his daughter, and our dog. I want a goat, and I want to name him **CAULIFLOWER!**

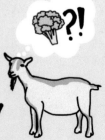

I do all my drawings on an iPad with an Apple pencil

Knowing what to expect makes cancer way easier.

(actually life is always easier when you know what happens next!)

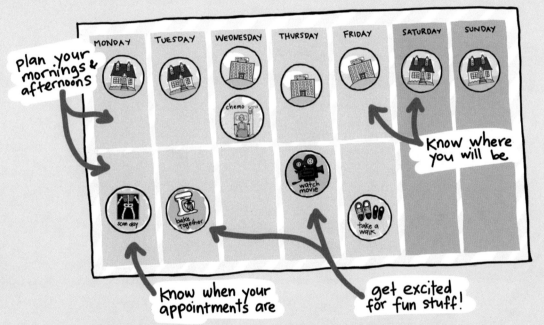

plan your mornings & afternoons

Know where you will be

know when your appointments are

get excited for fun stuff!

Change it up every week & take it from home to hospital!

find them at mightyandbright.com

(along with loads of other helpful stuff!)

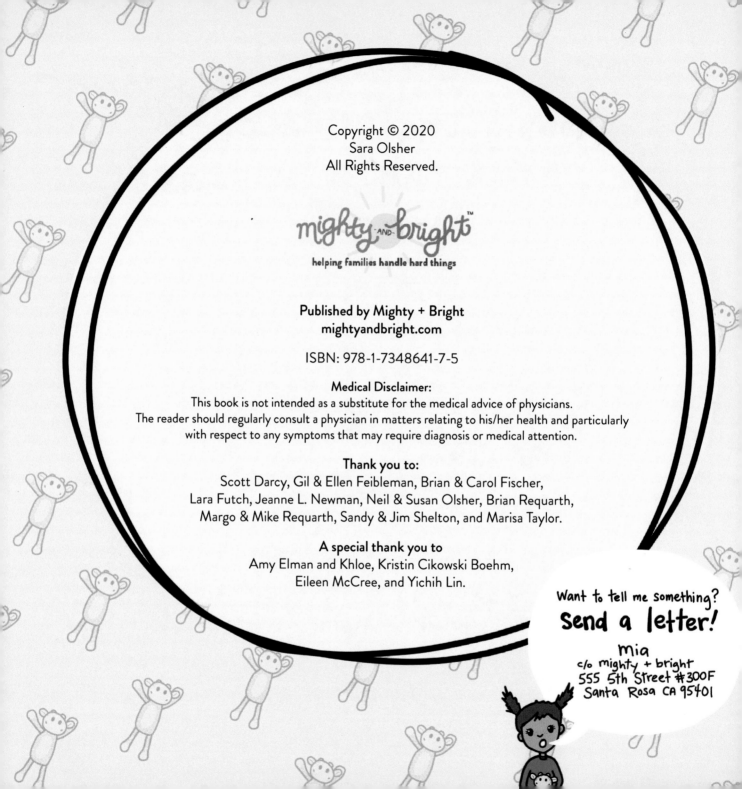

mighty -and- bright™

helping families handle hard things

Published by Mighty + Bright
mightyandbright.com

ISBN: 978-1-7348641-7-5

Medical Disclaimer:
This book is not intended as a substitute for the medical advice of physicians.
The reader should regularly consult a physician in matters relating to his/her health and particularly
with respect to any symptoms that may require diagnosis or medical attention.

Thank you to:
Scott Darcy, Gil & Ellen Feibleman, Brian & Carol Fischer,
Lara Futch, Jeanne L. Newman, Neil & Susan Olsher, Brian Requarth,
Margo & Mike Requarth, Sandy & Jim Shelton, and Marisa Taylor.

A special thank you to
Amy Elman and Khloe, Kristin Cikowski Boehm,
Eileen McCree, and Yichih Lin.

Want to tell me something?
send a letter!
mia
c/o mighty + bright
555 5th Street #300F
Santa Rosa CA 95401

Made in the USA
Coppell, TX
19 January 2022

71928170R00021